YOUR KNOWLEDGE HAS VALUE

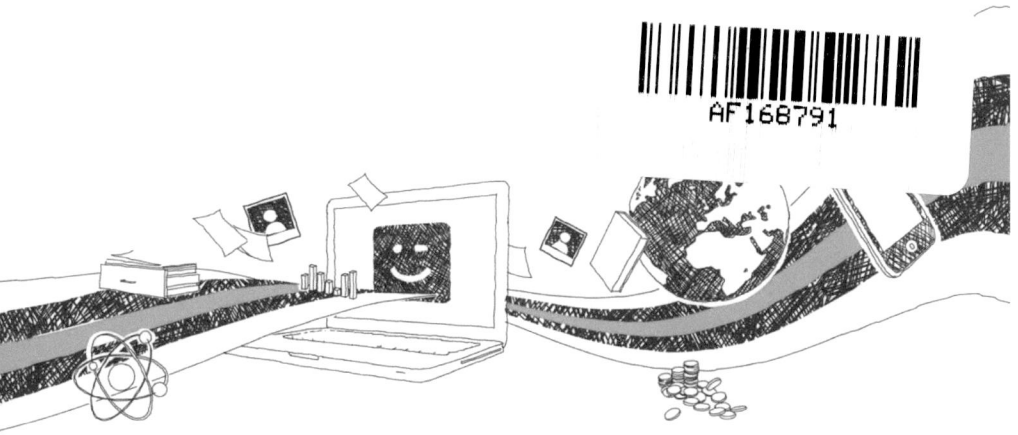

- We will publish your bachelor's and master's thesis, essays and papers

- Your own eBook and book - sold worldwide in all relevant shops

- Earn money with each sale

Upload your text at www.GRIN.com and publish for free

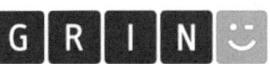

Bibliographic information published by the German National Library:

The German National Library lists this publication in the National Bibliography; detailed bibliographic data are available on the Internet at http://dnb.dnb.de .

This book is copyright material and must not be copied, reproduced, transferred, distributed, leased, licensed or publicly performed or used in any way except as specifically permitted in writing by the publishers, as allowed under the terms and conditions under which it was purchased or as strictly permitted by applicable copyright law. Any unauthorized distribution or use of this text may be a direct infringement of the author s and publisher s rights and those responsible may be liable in law accordingly.

Imprint:

Copyright © 2016 GRIN Verlag, Open Publishing GmbH
Print and binding: Books on Demand GmbH, Norderstedt Germany
ISBN: 9783668576896

This book at GRIN:

http://www.grin.com/en/e-book/381239/immune-thrombocytopenia-in-pregnancy

Patrick Kimuyu

Immune Thrombocytopenia in Pregnancy

GRIN Publishing

GRIN - Your knowledge has value

Since its foundation in 1998, GRIN has specialized in publishing academic texts by students, college teachers and other academics as e-book and printed book. The website www.grin.com is an ideal platform for presenting term papers, final papers, scientific essays, dissertations and specialist books.

Visit us on the internet:

http://www.grin.com/

http://www.facebook.com/grincom

http://www.twitter.com/grin_com

Immune Thrombocytopenia in Pregnancy

Name: Patrick K. Kimuyu

ABSTRACT

Thrombocytopenia occurs mostly in pregnant women, in which immune thrombocytopenia is believed to be one of the least prevalent forms of thrombocytopenia. Clinical studies indicate that immune thrombocytopenia occurs at a low rate of 11% compared to gestational thrombocytopenia, which occurs at a rate of 59%. However, it is characterized with moderate and severe thrombocytopenia with platelet counts decreasing below 100×10^9/L. Ordinarily, immune thrombocytopenia is caused by auto-immune reactions against platelets by anti-platelet antibodies, which destroy glycoprotein membranes forming platelet membranes.

Immune thrombocytopenia in pregnancy causes several risks to women and newborns. ITP pregnant women experience high risks of maternal hemorrhage compared to those suffering from other forms of thrombocytopenia. Despite the low percentage of ITP rates in pregnant women, extensive monitoring and management are required, primarily during prenatal care to reduce the risks associated with the disorder.

On the other hand, immune thrombocytopenia in pregnancy presents numerous neonatal concerns. The notion that, immune thrombocytopenia influences delivery alternatives has been disapproved by the recent clinical reports, which are based on randomized clinical trials. In the past, cesarean delivery was considered as a significant obstetric indication in ITP pregnant women. Currently, vaginal birth has been found to reduce trauma in newborns born of ITP mothers.

Moreover, treatment provided to immune thrombocytopenic women prior or during pregnancy causes neonatal concerns. For instance, splenectomy treatment prior to pregnancy has been found to increase free anti-platelet antibodies in maternal circulation, causing a significant risk of anti-platelet reactions in the fetus.

It has also been confirmed that, IgG anti-platelet antibodies are transferred from maternal circulation into the fetal body, and this may predispose the fetus to neonatal alloimmune thrombocytopenia (NAIT), leading to neonatal hemorrhage.

In conclusion, maternal and neonatal concerns associated with ITP can be reduced through platelet count monitoring during prenatal care.

IMMUNE THROMBOCYTOPENIA IN PREGNANCY

Thrombocytopenia occurs mostly in pregnant women, and they are characterized by a low platelet count. Platelet levels below $150 \times 10^9/l$ are associated with thrombocytopenia. However, thrombocytopenia is classified into three categories in accordance to the associated platelet level count. The main categories are mild, moderate and severe thrombocytopenia. In practice, pregnant women with platelet counts ranging between $100 - 150 \times 10^9/l$ are said to be suffering from mild thrombocytopenia while those who record platelet levels ranging between $50 - 100 \times 109/l$ suffer from moderate thrombocytopenia. Pregnant women whose platelet count decreases below $50 \times 109/l$ are said to be suffering from severe thrombocytopenia (Kam, Liew & Thompson, 2004).

It has been identified that, thrombocytopenia are caused by decreased platelet production in the patient's hematopoietic system. The second cause of thrombocytopenia is the accelerated destruction of platelets, primarily through autoimmune reactivity, owing to an autoimmune disorder. This condition has been found to be common in pregnant women with 10 percent of women experiencing thrombocytopenia (Kekomaki et al., 2000).

Immune thrombocytopenic purpura (ITP) is one of the most live-threatening forms of thrombocytopenia, and it is categorized as severe thrombocytopenia because it is characterized with platelet counts below $50 \times 10^9/l$. It occurs at a rate of 5 percent in pregnant women. McCrae and Stavrou (2009) report "immune thrombocytopenia (ITP) occurs in one or two of every 1,000 pregnancies, and accounts for 5% of cases of pregnancy-associated thrombocytopenia" (p. 2). Clinical research indicates that immune thrombocytopenia is caused by autoimmune reactions in the reticular endothelial system, in which platelet auto-antibodies destroy glycoprotein complexes forming the platelet membrane. As a result, platelet production in the reticular endothelial system decreases causing a significant decrease in platelet count in the circulatory system of the affected individual.

In most cases, immune thrombocytopenia causes a high risk of maternal hemorrhage. Therefore, treatment is required with extensive monitoring during the pre-natal and post-natal period to reduce the risks associated with the condition. However, it is worth noting that, immune thrombocytopenia causes minor risks on the newborn (Burstein et al. 2006).

Immune thrombocytopenia in pregnant women has been reviewed by researchers in the field of medicine to unravel the underlying mysteries related to the condition. In the last decade, several research studies advanced the clinical understanding on immune thrombocytopenia, and this has enhanced diagnosis, management and treatment approaches. For instance, immune thrombocytopenia was believed to cause significant risks on the infants who are born of immune thrombocytopenic women, but that issue has been clarified through advanced clinical trials (Cines & Blanchette, 2002). Currently, there is evidence that immune thrombocytopenia in pregnant women does not cause fatal risks to newborns.

In a clinical research study conducted, in 2005, by Burstein and his colleagues at Soroka University Medical Center, it was found out "there is a minor risk of thrombocytopenia in the newborn" (p. 2). This study was aimed at investigating obstetric risk factors, pregnancy outcomes and complications associated with immune thrombocytopenia in pregnant women. It studied the clinical implications of moderate to severe thrombocytopenia by comparing 199 pregnant participants whose platelet count levels were below $100 \times 10^9/l$, with 201 non-thrombocytopenia pregnant women. Their study included pregnant women who conceived between January 2003 to April 2004, and their methodology involved Mantel–Haenszel procedure (Burstein et al. 2006).

Clinical study results indicated that, immune thrombocytopenic women accounted for 11.05% of the study population while gestational thrombocytopenia was found to be the most common occurring form of thrombocytopenia with a total percentage of 59.3%. In regard to age of the participants, women without thrombocytopenia were found to be of younger ages compared to those suffering from thrombocytopenia. Their average age was estimated at 28 years while thrombocytopenic women recorded an age average of 30 years.

It was also identified that, immune thrombocytopenia was responsible for preterm deliveries, in which placental abruption occurred at higher rates in thrombocytopenic women than normal women. However, it is worth noting that, the high cases of preterm deliveries and placental abruption occurred after controlled labor induction, which was performed through the use of the Mantel–Haenszel procedure.

On the other hand, infants of thrombocytopenic women were recorded to have higher rates of Apgar scores, which were below 7 in 5 minutes, than infants born of non-thrombocytopenic women. Intra-uterine growth restriction was found to occur at a rate of 95 percent among thrombocytopenic women, in which women suffering from immune thrombocytopenia accounted for the highest percentage compared to those suffering from thrombotic thrombocytopenic purpura and anti-phospholipid antibodies (APLA) syndrome (Chehal et al.,2004). Conclusively, this research indicated that immune thrombocytopenia in women causes favorable perinatal complications compared to those suffering from HELLP syndrome and preeclampsia (Burstein et al. 2006).

The low prevalence of immune thrombocytopenia in pregnant women was also reaffirmed, in 2010, by a clinical study report released by the Cleveland Clinic Foundation. McCrae (2010) reported, "ITP is an uncommon cause of thrombocytopenia in pregnancy, occurring in between 1 in 1000 and 1 in 10,000 pregnant women as opposed to secondary ITP, which develops in association with viral infection" (p. 397). In addition, this study showed that an estimation of one-third of pregnancy-associated immune thrombocytopenia is diagnosed during pregnancy compared to two-thirds which is diagnosed first in non-pregnant women with preexisting diseases such as Human Immunodeficiency Virus (HIV), Helicobacter pylori and hepatitis c viral infection (McCrae, 2010).

On the other hand, immune thrombocytopenia has been found to become complicated during the third trimester of pregnancy, owing to a decrease in platelet count, primarily below 50x109/l, but most neonates record healthy outcomes. In a case study conducted in 2012, a woman with history of immune thrombocytopenia "delivered a healthy neonate with a platelet count of $125 \times 109/L$" (Gernsheimer, James & Stasi, 2012 p. 44).

In regard to the management of immune thrombocytopenia in pregnancy, it has been found out the mode of delivery among immune thrombocytopenic women does not depend on the condition. Instead, delivery modes in immune thrombocytopenic pregnant women should be based on obstetric indications. However, obstetric procedures, which increase hemorrhagic risk of the fetus such as vacuum extraction should be avoided (Gernsheimer, James & Stasi, 2012). In the past, immune thrombocytopenia in pregnant women was considered as a significant indication for cesarean delivery. However, recent clinical research reports do not indicate any significant association between immune thrombocytopenia with the modes of delivery among pregnant women suffering from the condition.

In contrast, investigators recommend the use of cesarean delivery in all pregnant women with history of immune thrombocytopenia. However, performing cesarean delivery is for the sake of the newborn, but not necessarily based on obstetric indications requiring safety measures to be observed to reduce the risk of the mother. This delivery is recommended for immune thrombocytopenic women to minimize to the newborns (Millar, 2012). In most cases, newborns delivered vaginally experience trauma during birth, and this raises a significant neonatal concern. Therefore, some investigators suggest that cesarean delivery can help to reduce trauma among newborns delivered by immune thrombocytopenic women.

In practice, these recommendations for performing cesarean delivery on immune thrombocytopenic women appear unrealistic. This was overruled after a comprehensive review of 474 newborns who were delivered by thrombocytopenic mothers using vaginal and cesarean deliveries. In this review, cesarean delivery was found to be associated with increased incidences of bleeding complications compared to vaginal delivery. Of the 474 newborns involved in the review, 30 % of newborns delivered by cesarean birth experienced bleeding complications compared to 29% of newborns delivered by vaginal birth. Millar (2012) remarks "Cesarean delivery has not been demonstrated to prevent bleeding complications in thrombocytopenic newborns" (par. 5).

Currently, there are numerous reviews, which have been published by different investigators on the issue of delivery modes among immune thrombocytopenic women, but most experts argue that none of these reviews bears substantial evidence over the case. For instance, Millar (2012) refutes the evidence provided by the currently published reviews comparing cesarean delivery and vaginal birth by stating "reviews published to date comparing vaginal birth to cesarean delivery in women with ITP are retrospective studies; none are randomized controlled trials" (par. 5). It is, therefore, necessary to reserve cesarean delivery for usual obstetric indications because there is no clear evidence on its benefit to neonates born of immune thrombocytopenic women.

In regard to neonatal concerns associated to immune thrombocytopenia, it has been found out that most medical approaches are based on the mother's safety, leaving the neonate at a risk. In the last decade, research studies produced controversial evidence on the safety of the newborns born of immune thrombocytopenic women. One of the most controversial neonatal concerns associated with immune thrombocytopenia was breastfeeding and the risk of experiencing auto-immune reactivity while developing in the maternal body. It is reported, "One trial evaluated the safety of breastfeeding in women with ITP, but there were no documentation of thrombocytopenia developing in any breastfed infants" (Millar, 2012 par. 2). Ordinarily, IgG antibodies are believed to cross placental membranes from maternal circulation into the fetal circulation during pregnancy. This biological phenomenon occurs to provide immunity to the fetus because; its reticular endothelial system is not developed to produce IgG antibodies for cell-mediated immune responses against pathogens. On the other hand, breast milk has been found to contain high levels of IgG antibodies, which are passed on to the infant through breastfeeding. Despite the an unprecedented evidence of auto-immune reactions in the newborns hematopoietic system, Millar (2012) advises that, platelet counts monitoring among breastfed newborns born of immune thrombocytopenic mothers serves a pivotal role in reducing the risk of autoimmune reactions, which may occur in the newborns' body. The fact that IgG anti-platelet antibodies are transmitted from immune thrombocytopenic mothers to their newborns through breast milk raises concerns of possible auto-immune reactions against platelets in the newborns circulation, and this may cause a significant decrease in neonatal platelet count. Therefore, it is necessary to monitor the newborn's platelets counts regularly as part of post-natal clinical procedures (Millar, 2012).

Despite the neonatal concern associated with breastfeeding, severe thrombocytopenia in newborns, which is caused by visceral or intracranial hemorrhage, is regarded to be the most fatal neonatal concern among newborns born of immune thrombocytopenic mothers (Rodeghiero et al., 2009). Therefore, the treatment provided to immune thrombocytopenic women should address this fatal neonatal concern.

In the past, it some investigators believed that splenectomy treatment on immune thrombocytopenic women prior to pregnancy reduced the newborn's risk of experiencing ant-platelets reactions during pregnancy. In contrast, recent clinical studies indicate that splenectomy serves as a risk factor for severe thrombocytopenia among newborns born of immune thrombocytopenic mothers who undergo splenectomy prior to pregnancy (Millar, 2012). It has been confirmed that splenectomy treatment on immune thrombocytopenic women prior to pregnancy increases the concentration of anti-platelet antibodies in the maternal circulation, owing to the removal of the spleen which destroys platelets and antibodies. Clinical screening programs have, so far, provided insight into the issue of severe immune thrombocytopenia in newborns born of immune thrombocytopenic mothers. Women with anti-platelet antibodies in their sera have been found to give birth to newborns with neonatal alloimmune thrombocytopenia (NAIT). Therefore, some investigators suggest that typing for platelet alloantigen during prenatal care may help in determining the risk of NAIT in newborns. However, prenatal screening for NAIT presents significant challenges because its clinical benefits have not been identified yet (ACOG, 1999).

However, diagnosis of severe thrombocytopenia in the fetus is accompanied with numerous difficulties. In the past, monitoring of the fetal platelet count was relatively impossible, but fetal scalp sampling has proved to be a reliable procedure for obtaining fetal platelet counts compared to cordocentesis procedure although they encompass difficulties during fetal platelet count sampling. This makes it difficult in determining severe thrombocytopenia in newborns born of immune thrombocytopenic mothers. Gernsheimer (2012) states, ""therapy late in gestation is generally based on the risk of maternal hemorrhage at delivery" (p. 201)

In general, immune thrombocytopenia is believed to be uncommon in pregnant women, but extensive understanding is required for designing the most appropriate clinical management approaches. McCrae and Stavrou state, "Though ITP is associated with a significant incidence of neonatal thrombocytopenia; it is generally not associated with major morbidity if properly managed" (p. 28).

REFERENCES

ACOG (1999). Thrombocytopenia in Pregnancy: Clinical Management Guidelines for Obstetrician- Gynecologists. *Int J Gynaecol Obstet.*, 67(2):117-28.

Burstein et al. (2006). Moderate To Severe Thrombocytopenia during Pregnancy. *European Journal of Obstetrics & Gynecology and Reproductive Biology*. Retrieved from http://www.medicine.wisc.edu/~williams/pregnancythrombocytopenia.pdf

Chehal, A. et al. (2004). Thrombotic Thrombocytopenic Purpura And Pregnancy: Reported Four Cases And Literature Review. *J Clin Apher*, 19:5–10.

Cines, D. & Blanchette, V. (2002). Immune Thrombocytopenic Purpura. *N Engl J Med.*, 346:13–25.

Gernsheimer, T. (2012). Thrombocytopenia in Pregnancy: Is This Immune Thrombocytopenia or…? *Hematology,* 2012(1): 198-202. doi: 10.1182/asheducation-2012.1.198

Gernsheimer, t., James, A. & Stasi, R. (2012). How I Treat Thrombocytopenia In Pregnancy. *Blood*, 121(1): 38-47. doi: 10.1182/blood-2012-08-448944

Kam, P., Liew, A. & Thompson, S. (2004). Review article, thrombocytopenia in the parturient. *Anaesthesia*, 59:255–64.

Kekomaki et al. (2000). Maternal Thrombocytopenia: A Population Based Study. *Acta Obstet Gynecol Scand*, 79:744–9.

McCrae, K. & Stavrou, E. (2009). Immune Thrombocytopenia in Pregnancy. *Hematol Oncol Clin Am.*, 23(6): 1-32. Retrieved from http://www.ncbi.nlm.nih.gov/pmc/articles/PMC2784425/

McCrae, K. (2010). *Thrombocytopenia in Pregnancy*. Retrieved from http://asheducationbook.hematologylibrary.org/content/2010/1/397.full

Millar, L. (2012). "*In Pregnancy, Treatment for ITP and NAIT Involves 2 Patients—the Mother and the Fetus.*" Retrieved from http://emedicine.medscape.com/article/208697-treatment#a1127

Rodeghiero, F. et al. (2009). Standardization of Terminology, Definitions and Outcome Criteria in Immune Thrombocytopenic Purpura of Adults and Children: Report from an International Working Group. *Blood*, 113(11):2386-2393.

YOUR KNOWLEDGE HAS VALUE

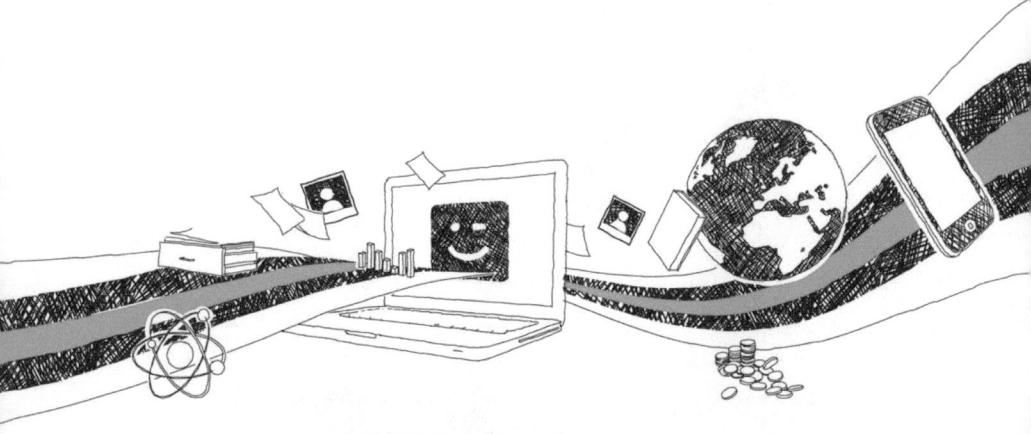

- We will publish your bachelor's and master's thesis, essays and papers

- Your own eBook and book - sold worldwide in all relevant shops

- Earn money with each sale

Upload your text at www.GRIN.com
and publish for free

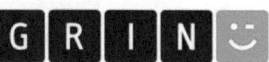